A Journey with Alzheimer's: A Caregiver's Memoir

Robert D. Thacker

Published by Summit Avenue Books, 2024.

Table of Contents

Chapter One: Sunny Days.. 1

Chapter Two: A Beautiful Life.......................................7

Chapter Three: Gathering Clouds 11

Chapter Four: Into the Unknown 19

Chapter Five: The Long Farewell..............................23

Chapter Six: Hopes for the Future 33

Chapter Seven: Legal Concerns................................37

Chapter Eight: Choosing a Care Facility 41

Chapter Nine: Working with Your Care Facility 45

Dedication

To Sylvia, whose love shines on in our hearts and our memories

Chapter One: Sunny Days

We met in 1954 in our early days of high school in Bruce County, Ontario, a rural community in Canada about a hundred miles northwest of Toronto. On our first double dates, we were paired with other people, she with my school buddy and I with her childhood friend. To be honest, I scarcely remember my date's name. She was a very nice girl, but she couldn't match the wit, cleverness and sunny outlook of her friend: Sylvia MacDuff, a vivacious brunette whose beauty sometimes earned comparisons to one of the popular young movie stars of that era, Elizabeth Taylor.

Sylvia and I met socially and danced many times over the next years, each dating people in our teen circle, but never each other. Still, that little glimmer of recognition, that sense of aligned stars, gleamed in the background for both of us.

After our graduation in 1956, I emigrated to the suburbs of Detroit, Michigan, determined to pursue a career in automobile design. Back in Ontario, Sylvia went to teachers' college in Toronto and was soon assigned to a two-room school near Wallaceburg, Ontario, where she boarded with her stepsister.

On a trip home to Bruce County in 1957 to visit my folks, I drove over to Sylvia's house to seek a date. My knock on the front door was answered by her mother, who explained that Sylvia was now living in Wallaceburg, adding that it was rather close to where I was now living. She mentioned that she was sure Sylvia would like to hear from me and gave me her number, the sly matchmaker! A weekend later, I made the eighty-minute drive for our first of many dates in the Wallaceburg area.

In 1958 Sylvia decided that teaching was not her heart's true calling. She returned home to Bruce County and took over bookkeeping and automotive parts managing in her stepfather's Ford dealership in Walkerton, where she flourished. We continued dating, now from a 200-mile distance, throughout the winter.

At the Easter break, we arranged for Sylvia and her friend Beth to visit Detroit and stay in a local motel, while Beth's fiancé stayed at the home where I boarded. On Good Friday evening, we four went to a drive-in movie where I interrupted the film to propose and present Sylvia with an engagement ring.

She said yes. I don't remember much about the movie, "GiGi," but I will forever treasure Sylvia's response!

We returned to Bruce County for our wedding at Walkerton United Church on October 17, 1959, both age 21. The long engagement was because she wanted a date that added her birthday and mine, June 11 and May 6.

We honeymooned in Ontario, New York, Pennsylvania and Washington D.C., before moving into our first apartment on the western edge of Detroit. She had completed her application for U.S. residency at the American embassy in Toronto, as had I in 1956. We had to wait three weeks for her green card to arrive so we could drive back up to Walkerton to retrieve our wedding gifts. For those three weeks we lived a rather spartan existence in our barely-furnished apartment.

In the happy years that followed, our family expanded. Our son Gregg was born in 1960 and our daughter Shelly three years later. In 1962 we moved into our first house in Livonia, Michigan, and I started my first of 37 years at the Ford Design Center in Dearborn. We enjoyed good health, wonderful family vacations, and made many life-long friends in our neighborhood and at Ford. We had our share of arguments and disagreements as one can expect with two strong-willed and intelligent adults, but we always managed to resolve them. We also managed to raise our two children to become high achievers and our two granddaughters are well along the same path. This was not an easy accomplishment given the wild and free sixties and seventies when opportunities to go off the rails abounded.

In 1974 we moved ten miles west to Northville, Michigan, where we would live until our retirement.

During those busy years while we were raising our children, Sylvia also continued her education and became a Registered Nurse. She worked in local hospitals, then joined the nursing staff at a doctor's office, which she enjoyed until the doctor moved to Arizona and she disliked the standards of the one who replaced her. After a few months as a stay-at-home mom, she agreed to take on a nursing management position at a nursing home owned by our family dentist. She discovered that she loved caring for the elderly and spent the remainder of her nursing career there.

Soon, our children left the nest and married, happily pursuing their own goals, and Sylvia's mind raced ahead to the next challenge...one inspired by fond memories of enjoying afternoon tea with friends in her youth.

She meticulously planned and opened a Victorian restaurant called The Sweet Afton Tea Room in the historic Old Village district of Plymouth, Michigan in 1988. Her menu included high tea, scones and shortbread, cucumber sandwiches and shepherd's pie, all served in a charming atmosphere that was authentic in every detail, right down to the English porcelain tea pots and cups and a vintage cash register that rang up in British pence. Named after her favorite poem by Scottish poet Robert Burns, Sweet Afton earned rave reviews from customers and the local media alike, and the *Detroit News* recognized it as one of the top ten restaurants in the entire Metro Detroit area.

The years ahead were satisfying but extremely busy as she enjoyed building her business and making many lasting friendships. In 1996 she decided she was ready to retire from the daily work of running a restaurant, so she sold Sweet Afton to one of her many devoted customers.

Within just a few months, however, she grew tired of being retired.

So she launched into planning yet another career change. The new owners of Sweet Afton had moved the tea room to downtown Plymouth, where there was more foot traffic, which left the original location in the historic Old Village vacant. Sylvia rented the original space a second time and opened a new shop: The Canadian Bakery. In addition to selling baked goods inspired by her cherished family recipes, she also developed a side venture catering in-home tea parties, which became popular for birthdays. She continued operating The Canadian Bakery until her second retirement—and my first—in April 1999.

For the first time since our arrival in Michigan forty years earlier, we left the Detroit area and headed north, moving into a beach house with a picturesque view of Lake Huron. After the move, Sylvia found herself feeling anxious and unsettled, and she went to see a counselor, who suggested she needed some new occupations for her ever-curious and active mind. The counselor encouraged her to apply to Mensa, the international organization for people with high I.Qs. She passed the entrance exam and was accepted. We attended many of their social events in the years that followed. She also began to collect owls, the Mensa mascot.

Sylvia's lifelong love of gardening led her to the Iosco County Master Gardener program, where she became certified and earned credits for leading a class of residents in a local nursing home, teaching them to grow seedlings and house plants. As always, she loved working with the elderly and sat with them for many hours, listening to their life stories.

Around this time, one of Sylvia's friends suffered a traumatic experience: her husband became so ill that he required nursing home care, and the friend lost almost her entire life savings and everything she owned paying for it. Sylvia did not want the same fate to befall us. She insisted that we find a way to avoid losing everything we had worked so hard to earn. So in 2012, while we were both still healthy, we met with a local elder-law attorney and drew up a trust.

We had always agreed that we would care for each other at home for as long as possible, even if one of us fell seriously ill. But we also agreed that neither of us wanted to become such a burden to the other that it endangered their well-being. We would have professional nursing care take over if necessary.

The legal structure of our trust established that if one of us were forced to go into a nursing home, a court case would be filed to separate our finances, and the ill person would become eligible for support by Michigan Health and Human Services. The ill spouse would become a legal dependent of the well spouse, who the court would direct to manage the ill person's finances and all of their life and medical decisions.

The trust we signed that day would go on to save us a substantial portion of our nest egg, funds that may be required for my care in the future. I thank God for Sylvia's foresight. The reality of life expectancy has most wives out-living their husbands, so I viewed the trust as providing for her financial stability when she survived me.

But that wasn't how things turned out.

Chapter Two: A Beautiful Life

Little is known about what causes Alzheimer's disease. Sylvia and I were born just before the outbreak of World War II and I don't remember even hearing the word in my youth.

I was raised on a farm while Sylvia spent her early years in a small industrial city. Our families were poor by modern standards, but our meager finances were quite common at that time, during the lingering aftermath of the Great Depression.

Sylvia's father enlisted in the Canadian military and was mostly absent from the time she was about three years old. He was later injured, met a volunteer woman in the hospital, and abandoned Sylvia and her mother by war's end. He married his mistress and moved out west, raising two daughters whom he fervently protected from learning of his prior life and fatherhood. He never made any of the court-ordered payments to support his firstborn daughter.

As a result, Sylvia's mother faced life as a single parent and a divorced woman, a status that still carried shame in the 1940s. She was also forced to find work, which resulted in Sylvia's further neglect. Sylvia was often unclean when she went to school and left alone at a very young age until her mother returned home from her job. Her mother also became a lifelong heavy smoker.

When Sylvia was nine, her mother remarried and they moved to a larger town and out of the abject poverty of her childhood. Sylvia's surname also changed, from Duke to MacDuff.

The traumatic and deliberate abandonment by her biological father affected Sylvia all of her life. After our marriage, she spent years in sessions with psychiatrists and managed to lead a normal day-to-day existence. But the suffering, anxiety, and fear of abandonment lingered just below the surface. After our children were born in the 1960s, Sylvia launched a search for her father, longing for a renewed connection, or at least a little kindness from the man who had turned his back on her when she was only three. She found his phone number. She made contact.

And he rejected her all over again. He was terrified that his shameful past would be revealed to his second family, who revered him as a fine, upstanding husband and father. He refused any reunion with Sylvia or any contact with his two grandchildren. He didn't even want to see their photographs.

Given the chance to redeem himself, he proved once again to be a dismal failure as a parent and a human being.

This second rejection was devastating for Sylvia. She spun into a downward spiral, physically and emotionally. From then on, any rejection she experienced in life had an overwhelming negative impact on her. Her fear of the pain of rejection filled her with a need to excel to avoid it.

I don't know if early trauma may help sow the seeds of Alzheimer's years later. I just know that Sylvia went through hell in her childhood. Only through immense effort was she able to overcome the lifelong, cruel abandonment by her biological father. Thanks to her deep faith, grit, intelligence and determination, she managed to earn two college degrees, create a loving family, and pursue fulfilling careers as a teacher, registered nurse, business owner, and community volunteer. She took the pain of her childhood and transformed it into a beautiful life, making her an exemplary success story.

Then a disease called Alzheimer's came to steal it all away, piece by piece.

Chapter Three: Gathering Clouds

I hate the term *dementia*, often used interchangeably with Alzheimer's. The very sound of the word *dementia* implies madness instead of the reality of this illness: a physical disability of the brain to convey messages to the rest of the body.

Alzheimer's arrived in subtle ways and slowly shredded the beautiful life Sylvia and I had shared for sixty years.

My first awareness that something was wrong began in 2010, when Sylvia was 72 years old. She started to have some uncharacteristically angry outbursts, with no clear cause. At social gatherings, she would sometimes express inappropriate remarks to friends, seeming to have forgotten the norms of polite restraint in conversation. Mood-swings, forgetfulness and social anxiety soon emerged and slowly progressed to ever deeper issues.

She had always enjoyed keeping a diary and wrote many journals of our noteworthy travels and adventures. They are a treasure to me now. One notebook from 2014 is titled *Memory Journal*. In it, she started writing down family history along with names of friends and events. She was already aware of her declining memory, and was making an effort to capture everything and everyone she loved before she forgot them.

In 2014 our doctor diagnosed Sylvia with thyroid problems and suggested treatment. We thought perhaps that could be contributing to her memory troubles and declining health. She was referred to a surgeon who removed most of her para-thyroid glands. During her post-op recovery in a local hospital, she complained to me about unsanitary treatment by nurses' aides the night before. She was overwrought with anxiety about it.

Our doctor said it never happened. She had imagined the whole thing.

That was my first concrete signal that something was going drastically wrong. After her discharge, it was a long drive home, though only 60 miles.

During 2015 she still drove her car, read books, shopped, cooked and cleaned. She wrote notes to remind herself of upcoming events and appointments and jotted down phone conversations.

By 2016, however, her desire to go out in public, get washed and dressed, drive or shop began to decline. I had to work hard to get her to the doctor or medical lab for checkups. During her annual physical in 2017, her doctor administered a cognitive test. She was subsequently diagnosed as having Alzheimer's disease.

It wasn't easy hearing that word, and yet it wasn't a total shock. The doctor and staff gave me a little information but were unable to suggest any treatments that might help. There simply aren't any effective treatments for this all-too-common illness. I asked if a dietary supplement such as Prevagen might be worth a try. The doctor told me to save my money. I turned to the internet and gathered what little information I could find from medical websites. The hardest fact to accept was that life expectancy from the time of diagnosis is typically just five to ten years.

The final two entries in Sylvia's *Memory Journal* are dated July 16 and 17, 2017...but there are no notes written beneath either date. In just three short years, she had lost her ability to hold onto her memories long enough to write them down.

I gradually took over managing all her medications and healthcare appointments along with all the shopping, cooking, checking accounts, cleaning and laundry. I still have the last greeting cards she bought and gave me for my birthday, Father's Day and Christmas in 2017.

In 2018 her driver's license came up for renewal, but it would have required her to go to the Department of Motor Vehicles and fill out a questionnaire. She had not driven for many months and said she couldn't take the test, so we let her license expire.

I had one of our bathrooms remodeled to make it easier and more secure for her to use, adding grab bars and a zero-entry shower with a chair. She used the shower chair one time, but I never convinced her to try it again. She preferred to use the sink and a washcloth for bathing.

She lost interest in contacting friends she used to enjoy chatting with. Gradually, she stopped using the phone altogether.

Long-ago memories became more vivid to her. She asked when her parents or mine were coming to visit. Each time, I gently told her that they had all passed away. She started asking constant questions about more recent events—the same questions repeated over and over.

By mid-2018, it became difficult to leave her alone for even a short time. She could still use the landline, but couldn't manage a cell phone. She could use the TV selector, but not the DVD player. To soothe her nerves when I had to run an errand, I made oversized flash cards with large printing on them stating where I was and my cell number. I set up a little card with clock hands showing when I would return. Still, every time I came home, she would ask where I had been. Her ability to understand information, whether written or spoken, was declining day by day.

She stopped playing the piano, a favorite activity since childhood.

She was still able to use the restroom independently and get snacks and her favorite A&W Root Beer from the kitchen. Unknown to me, she had stopped oral hygiene.

We began to sleep in separate bedrooms so that we could each get some rest, since I had always been a heavy snorer and she had begun waking several times a night. One night, I woke to the sound of her urgently shouting my name. I leaped out of bed and rushed to her room, only to become light-headed and fall to the floor. In just a few seconds I was conscious and able to console her, but the image of my "demise" was etched on her mind—and she refused to ever sleep in that bedroom again.

She adopted a love seat in the kitchen as her preferred place to be, a sunny corner where she could watch TV or enjoy the view of the lake. She began to spend all her time there, day and night. Even for her five-foot stature, the love seat was not a comfortable place to sleep. I tried various pillows and wedge cushions, but she just wanted it as it was. She slept there with her feet resting against the bottom bolster and her neck on the top bolster with pillows to fill in. I suggested we get a hospital bed but she scoffed at the idea. She preferred the love seat.

By the summer of 2019, it was becoming more and more difficult to get her to leave the house at all. I managed to get her to the medical lab seven miles away for bloodwork and a visit with her doctor. A few weeks later, part of her upper bridgework came out. Fortunately, it didn't cause her any pain. With great effort, I got her to the dentist for an examination and cleaning. X-rays showed extensive neglect and he urged oral surgery—but that would have required spending two or three days in a city 65 miles away. I knew she would never be able to handle that, and she agreed. There would be no oral surgery.

A few weeks later, she had a fall off the love seat and I couldn't get her up from the floor. I called EMS. The paramedics transported her to the hospital in an ambulance. After taking X-rays, the doctors said she hadn't broken any bones but they diagnosed her with a urinary tract infection (UTI). When she was discharged, I had the ambulance return her home to the familiar comfort of her love seat.

With winter coming on, I could no longer get her safely out of the house to the car for any appointments, so I engaged the services of the Visiting Physicians Association. They were able to conduct doctor visits, lab work, X-rays, and even echocardiograms right in our home. I still had confidence that I was giving her the care she needed.

By the end of 2019, she was still able to get up and walk around the house, use the bathroom independently, and converse with me in complete sentences. She still had a good appetite as long as I cut up her food for her.

And then 2020 arrived.

It had been three years since her Alzheimer's diagnosis and we were struggling daily with its ungodly demands. By March, she was eating less and less and could no longer use the restroom. I bought incontinence supplies and washed constant loads of laundry. By July, she was growing weaker and walking less and less. It took major effort just to get her up to sit in a chair while I changed her bedding.

It felt agonizing to watch as she died a little bit every week. She had deteriorated from a brilliant, vivacious, outgoing woman and Mensa member to a shut-in unable to speak a complete sentence. It was a test of our Christian faith which we had shared for more than sixty years.

One morning in July, she was standing beside me while I changed her bedding when she suddenly said, "Oh, my knees!" and fell to the floor. I called EMS and they once again took her to the emergency room for tests. She passed a CT scan but was—once again—diagnosed with a UTI. She spent two days in the hospital to treat the UTI, during which a physical therapist evaluated her.

This time, the hospital discharge and placement officer suggested that she should go to a nursing home. I reluctantly agreed, if she would get physical therapy there. I hoped that some PT might restore her ability to walk again, and then she could return home.

Unfortunately, our insurance company refused payment for PT because she hadn't been cooperative with the hospital's physical therapist. It was infuriating that they didn't take into account her Alzheimer's diagnosis and her fear of falling again. I told the discharge staff to call an ambulance to take her home, and I would have the Visiting Physicians Association set up additional in-home care and PT.

Back at home, she refused to eat. She asked what was wrong with her and I told her again that she had Alzheimer's. For the first time, she asked if it was fatal.

"We're all going to die," I told her, "but not for a long time."

She replied, "I just want to die."

Her words stunned me and filled me with despair. I had never heard her speak that way before. She also told me that I was a good man and she loved me. Those words, at least, gave me some solace.

For a few brief days, we resumed our life as it had been before the latest hospital visit. She slept on the love seat. I did endless loads of laundry. Tried to persuade her to eat. Prayed that I could get her the help she needed. It took a week before the VPA doctor came. To my relief and gratitude, she ordered PT, visiting nurses, and a hospital bed. With her help, Sylvia got up and sat while her bedding was changed and I bathed her.

Unfortunately, it would take another seven days before the visiting nurses or PT could be scheduled. During that week, I could not get Sylvia up from the love seat at all. I was able to help her roll to the side while I changed absorbent pads and cleaned her as well as I could. But when the physical therapist finally arrived and we got her to move, he was appalled to see the beginnings of bedsores. He strongly suggested I take her back to the hospital.

I called EMS—again—on July 25th, 2020.

Watching the paramedics wheel her out on a gurney, I felt overwhelmed with sorrow, afraid that this might be the last time she ever saw home.

Chapter Four: Into the Unknown

We had reached the point I had dreaded since Sylvia's health began to decline ten years before: despite our promises to each other, I was no longer able to provide the care she needed in our home.

After she spent a night in the hospital for treatment and observation, the hospital discharge officer strongly recommended she be moved to a long-term care facility. With great reluctance and sadness, I agreed. She was transferred to a local nursing home about twenty minutes north of our house. Because this was during the height of the Covid pandemic, no visitors were allowed inside, not even to ease the transition for a new arrival. I could only follow in my car as the ambulance transported Sylvia from the hospital. I was forced to say goodbye outside the entrance, praying that this was the right place for her.

The Tawas area had four nursing facilities to choose from, each with about 50 resident rooms and areas for physical therapy, recreational activities and dining. One was a large residence with accommodations for patients ranging from minimal care to full care, while the other three were smaller, private nursing homes. Unfortunately, due to the Covid restrictions, I was unable to tour inside any of the facilities; however, I had visited friends in each of them over the years and had formed opinions about their quality.

One facility had a memory-care wing, which was a negative for me. I had visited once at lunch time and the dining room was chaotic, with only one attendant for about every 7 patients, which made it impossible to control the more aggressive

Alzheimer's patients. At other facilities I had visited, where memory-care residents are mixed in with the general population, the aggressiveness common to some Alzheimer's patients was tempered by resistance from the non-Alzheimer's patients, which created a more peaceful environment.

My favorite of the four options was one I'll call the Manor, and my good opinion was reinforced by our son Gregg and his wife Kathy, who had just spent six years caring long-distance for her ailing parents in Florida. Gregg and Kat liked that the Manor offered large, single-resident rooms with big windows. Another plus was the shared ensuite bathroom, open only to the adjacent patient's room. Sylvia was unable to get out of bed, so her shared bathroom became private for her neighbor. In comparison to their Florida experiences, Gregg and Kat said the Manor looked fantastic. In the days ahead, I was pleased to find that the Manor's care was consistently clean, thorough and loving.

The Manor filed and won an appeal so that our private health insurance paid for Sylvia's stay, including daily physical therapy. However, with her loss of appetite and weakening muscle condition, they were never able to get her to stand or walk on her own during those first few weeks. Consequently, her case was shifted to private-pay as of August 17, because it was evident that Sylvia was going to require full-time nursing care from then on.

I realized that it was time to call our elder-law attorney. I informed her of the situation and asked her to proceed with the legal processes of the trust we had created in 2012. Meanwhile, I began to pay almost $9,000 per month to the Manor and filed a claim to receive the $130 per day reimbursement provided under our long-term care insurance policy, which we had been paying into since 1995.

To establish that Sylvia was eligible for Michigan Health and Human Services (MHHS) status under our trust, it was necessary to prepare and schedule a court case. I would need to appear before a judge in the jurisdiction where she now resided, Iosco County. It took about three months to get on the county court's schedule, and the date was set for October 2020.

My contribution to the case involved supplying hundreds of financial, medical and legal documents. Our attorney showed me one of her other case files, which was a stack of papers about the size of an old Sears catalogue! It was an extremely busy time for me, balancing visits with Sylvia with deep searches for long-forgotten fragments of our legal and medical history.

Thanks to his recent experience with his in-laws, our son Gregg was able to help guide and support me through the process. Finally, after many meetings with the law firm and approval of our diligent efforts to provide the necessary data, we were ready for the court appearance. Covid pandemic control measures were still in place, so the hearing took place via Zoom. Gregg and I went to the attorney's office in Saginaw and she linked us virtually to the judge and his officials in his Iosco County courtroom.

I will always be grateful for the expertise of our elder-care attorney. Thanks to her careful preparation, the hearing went smoothly. The court found Sylvia dependent upon me and appointed me her legal guardian. They appointed MHHS as her main financial support, with a modest co-pay from her bank account, which I would manage. Our attorney informed MHHS that we had long-term care insurance, but they told her they would not be utilizing that coverage as part of Sylvia's financing. (According to our attorney, this policy is different in some other states.) The long-term care insurance company reimbursed me for the full amount of all my payments to the nursing home, along with a modest per-diem for each day since her Alzheimer's diagnosis that I had provided her care at home.

It was a tremendous relief to have the financial aspects of Sylvia's care settled. If not for our trust, we could have lost everything, because we still had a long road ahead.

Chapter Five: The Long Farewell

Because of the pandemic-control measures in place across the state of Michigan during Covid, visitors were forbidden to set foot inside the nursing home. To see my wife of more than 60 years, I could only stand or sit outside her window. I had been Sylvia's voice and advocate throughout the four years since her diagnosis—by her side for every doctor's appointment, every hospital stay, every emergency room visit. I shuddered to think of her being helpless now, deprived of my assistance, unable to communicate with healthcare workers who could not understand her needs. Our forced separation felt like a prison sentence.

I set up a tall, portable chair to enable me to sit outside her window, and we managed to improvise a way to communicate through the glass. Our son Gregg found a baby monitor on Amazon that did the trick. The base was placed in Sylvia's room, and the nursing home staff simply had to plug it in and turn it on so we could talk. She didn't need to press any keys to speak; I pressed the key on my monitor to speak and released it to listen.

She no longer spoke in sentences and became extremely frustrated if her single-word responses weren't understood. I visited outside her window daily, then returned home to cry over what we had lost. It felt like mourning, a long farewell to a loved one who was still in this world yet no longer fully present. I was resolved to accept the fact that she had twenty-four-hour care now, better than what I or home care could provide. But I was haunted that I couldn't hold her hand to reassure her of my love and caring. I knew that she must feel abandoned by my absence in her daily life, and abandonment had always been her greatest fear.

One Sunday, I dreamed that Sylvia was home, that she dressed up and went for a walk with me in the neighborhood. She even called a friend on the phone. Then I awoke and discovered that it was only a cruel illusion. I wondered if she dreamed anymore, hoping that dreams, at least, might provide a pleasant escape for her. When I asked her that afternoon, she said she had no recollection of any dreams. This ugliest of ailments had robbed her of not only her memories, but dreams, fantasy, whimsy, creativity or any enjoyable diversions. She could no longer remember her cat, Sweetie Pie, or our home, or any close friends.

In October 2020, the state finally relaxed its Covid prevention rules for nursing homes just a bit, enough to allow face-to-face visits—provided they took place outdoors, that everyone stayed at least six feet apart, and that the facility provided weather protection. A small facility like the Manor couldn't afford to meet such rules. Consequently, I still visited through her window, though the cool, wet weather of fall restricted the regularity and length of our visits. I wished the facility could use an empty room as a visiting area, but that was not allowed.

By November, indoor face-to-face visits were finally allowed. Sylvia was lifted into a wheelchair and rolled down to what had previously been the communal dining room, now deserted. It had been four months since we had been allowed to be in the same room. But we could only meet across the length of a six-foot table, with a Certified Nursing Assistant (CNA) sitting 15 feet away, both of us wearing masks, not permitted to touch.

This arrangement lasted only one week before Covid numbers spiked and nursing homes went into lockdown again. Visitors were once more forbidden to set foot indoors. I was back to standing outside her window in the cold and talking via the baby monitor.

All too soon, Michigan's winter moved in with icy determination. The rapidly dropping temperatures made it nearly impossible to sit or stand outside her window for more than a few minutes. I bought good old-fashioned long underwear and an electrically-heated vest. Despite repeated explanations of why I couldn't come inside, she was unable to understand. At Christmas, our children, grandchildren and I sent presents and cards to be delivered to her. Sylvia showed signs of enjoying them, as I stood outside in the freezing cold and snow, trying to help her understand who the items were from.

In January 2021, a blizzard blanketed our area with 12 inches of snow and sub-zero temperatures. My visits became limited to days with temperatures above 25 degrees Fahrenheit, and then only for a maximum of about 15 minutes. I got permission from the care facility to pull my 4-wheel drive car through the snowbank near her room, so I could visit from inside the vehicle, parked ten feet from her window. She could see and hear me using our baby monitor, but I couldn't see her due to the bright sun reflecting on her window. This solution worked for a while, until the increasing snow built up and I feared my car would get stuck in the snowbank.

On February 14, I stood outside the cold window and described the cards and gifts we had all sent her for Valentines' Day. A very considerate CNA read the cards, and Sylvia smiled and joked with her. This was one of the few high points of our visits that winter.

By late February, indoor visits were once again allowed, but with the same set-up as before: in the empty dining room, six-foot table between us, no touching, everyone masked. She was clearly uncomfortable being away from the familiar confines of her own room. We would visit for the allowed 30 minutes, then she wanted to get back to her comfort zone. During one visit, I became aware that she thought I was there to take her home! In the end, as the nurse paused for us to say goodbye, I saw anguish on her face at our parting. I had to walk away with a heavy heart, and cried myself home, wondering why God had allowed one of His wonderful and compassionate servants to be so degraded by this cruel, brain-malfunctioning illness.

The rules for visitors seemed to change on an almost weekly basis as Covid cases abated and then resurged. Most days I was able to visit inside, but on other occasions I would be banished to stand outside her window again.

Thankfully, when Covid vaccines became available in the spring of 2021, nursing home residents were at the top of the priority list. As the pandemic finally began to recede, I was at last allowed to visit Sylvia in her room.

I began a new routine of visiting in her room almost every day for two or more hours. She had always loved chocolate, so I kept a supply of Kit-Kat bars and Hershey's kisses in the drawer of her dresser, which I gave to her during our visits. And I always kept a 12-pack of her favorite A&W Zero Sugar Root Beer in the fridge of the nutrition room, so the CNAs could bring one to her each day. She enjoyed those through a straw.

Sometimes they would wheel her to the dining room and I would go along to assist her. Fun group activities like bingo were once again being offered, but Sylvia could no longer participate in any activity that required memory, even puzzles. Her lifelong love of reading had also been stolen by Alzheimer's. On a few occasions, I took her outdoors in her wheelchair to look at flowers and enjoy some fresh air; however, she always thought I was taking her home and became very sad when we had to return inside.

I bought a compact DVD player and we repeatedly watched every episode of her favorite PBS shows like "Doc Martin" and "All Creatures Great and Small." She also showed some interest in classic movies featuring her favorite stars like Montgomery Clift and Elizabeth Taylor.

Music was a particular comfort to her. I brought in her portable CD player and played big band music, 1950s pop hits, and classical and piano concertos for her. She especially enjoyed Canadian entertainer Leonard Cohen's two-hour London performance, listening to it over and over, becoming very engaged in the music. She would move her hands in time to the tempo and smile and say, "I love you."

At the holidays, we would watch Christmas movies and she would sing along to old carols and hymns from long ago—and even when the scene changed in the movie, she would continue singing every stanza of the carol, recalling the words perfectly. It's one of the many mysteries of Alzheimer's, that music stayed with her long after she had lost so many other memories.

Understandably, the staff rarely played her music, so she had to make do with TV or radio for the twenty-plus hours I wasn't there. The TV had basic cable service but she wasn't able to use the remote very well. She could only click up the list until it was stuck on the jewelry auction, where it would stay until my arrival at one o'clock the next afternoon.

In July of 2021, after we were all fully vaccinated, our daughter, her husband and our two granddaughters were able to visit from Minnesota. Under the Covid rules that summer, only two visitors were allowed in the room at one time. Sylvia was in good spirits, but sadly she no longer remembered her grandchildren. She did show a spark of recognition of our daughter Shelly, a writer: she couldn't recall her name, but repeatedly said, "The words...the words" as she looked at her with love. She also couldn't recall the name of our son-in-law, Mark, who had always been the family comedian...but she smiled when he walked in and said warmly, "the funny guy!" We all felt blessed to be able to gather again as a family after a year and a half apart.

Throughout her time at the Manor, Sylvia's physical health had remained stable. Her vital signs and moderate food intake stayed pretty much the same month to month, and she had no recurrence of the UTIs that had plagued her for years. She was able to handle utensils and cups and could eat and drink independently.

In the summer of 2023, the Manor re-introduced performances by local musicians. Sylvia especially liked one talented guitar player who sang songs popular with those of us in our eighties. He visited every two weeks and played in the dining room. All the residents, including Sylvia, got into the beat, tapping their toes, clapping their hands and singing along. It was great to see her enjoy the lively performances. It brought back memories of the vivacious girl I had fallen in love with more than 60 years before.

But by that autumn, her health began to decline. She stopped eating for several weeks. She even refused the chocolates she had always loved. She lost more than 30 pounds. The nurses, doctor and I were concerned. The social service director suggested that it was time to bring in hospice care.

It was devastating to hear that word. *Hospice* in my mind meant *end of life*. In that moment, I knew Sylvia's long years of struggle with Alzheimer's were nearing their inevitable conclusion. I gave my approval for her to receive hospice care. It was a long drive home and a frightful night for me.

Thankfully, she was able to stay in her familiar room at the Manor, now under the care of the hospice team instead of the regular nursing staff. The goal of hospice care was to make her as comfortable as possible. There would be no more trips to the hospital, no emergency resuscitation measures used, and they discontinued a couple of the medications she had been prescribed in the past, such as the drug to lower her cholesterol.

The hospice team provided an air mattress that gave her comfortable support in bed, and they introduced a fully adjustable wheelchair that fit her much better and was more maneuverable. Their nursing and counseling were impeccable and much appreciated. I was especially grateful for the kindness, prayers and support of the hospice chaplain.

During one of his visits, the chaplain told me that I was a legend. Surprised, I asked him to explain.

"That's how the whole staff here thinks of you," he said. "You visited outside Sylvia's window in rain, snow, and freezing weather for months, and you've visited in her room almost daily since then. It's been almost four years."

I never thought I was being "legendary," just a faithful and dutiful husband. Our oldest granddaughter once asked me how I could cope with the stress of being a caregiver, and I told her I considered it my duty as a husband, "in sickness and in health."

A couple of years later, driving home from college, that same granddaughter said to her mom, "When I get married someday, I want a man who loves me as much as Grandpa loves Grandma."

That's a legend I can live with. I hope I get to meet that God-sent man before I die.

When Sylvia had been placed under hospice care, the team had explained that the typical life expectancy for hospice patients is about six months. But by late November, she seemed to rally. Her appetite returned, she enjoyed chocolate again, and she regained 15 pounds. She was cheerful and smiled with her caregivers and with me. She couldn't form many words anymore but she could still say "I love you."

During the Christmas season, she became subdued and didn't find much joy in presents, holiday décor, visits from our family, or her favorite carols and hymns.

After Christmas, her appetite vanished again. She took only a few bites at each meal. She mumbled but formed few recognizable words. One day she distinctly said, "I'm going to die." I tried to reassure her, telling her that she was being cared for in the healing arms of our Savior.

On January 16, she managed to say, "I love you" and went to sleep. I returned home to eat dinner, feeling anxious about her condition. I went to bed to read a book and try to sleep, but at

9:30 p.m., the Manor called to say that Sylvia's breathing was in great distress. I dressed and rushed to her side.

They had put her on oxygen, but the effort to breathe was wracking her whole body. The hospice team was called in. I played her favorite piano music softly on her CD player. As midnight passed, I held her hand, whispering my love and my prayers. I knew she was near the end, and I wanted her to know she wasn't alone. I prayed that God would ease her passage from this earth.

She stopped breathing. The hospice nurse and CNAs joined our prayers.

At 12:14 a.m. on January 17, 2024, Sylvia released her last breath in a final gentle puff as she passed into the arms of Jesus. Her agonizing struggle with the horrors of Alzheimer's had reached its merciful end. She was at peace at last.

Chapter Six: Hopes for the Future

I was not aware of the many implications of Alzheimer's disease when Sylvia was first diagnosed, and not much more enlightened about this mysterious ailment by the end. I spent nine years searching the internet, seeking answers to how it progresses, what are the stages, what are the types, what I could do to help her. For patients and caregivers alike, there are too many questions and too few answers.

I got some basic information from the diagnosing doctor and a recommendation to reach out to the Alzheimer's Association of America. My own doctor's staff printed out information about support groups and elder organizations in my area. However, we had retired to a beach house located between two small towns twenty miles apart, and our home is sixty miles from the nearest small city. During the four plus years I cared for Sylvia at home, I couldn't risk leaving her alone in the evenings while I took a long drive to a distant caregiver meeting.

Unfortunately, most Alzheimer's resources and support groups are concentrated near large cities; they're rare or non-existent in rural areas. Consequently, I was pretty much on my own. I tried online support groups but found it difficult to connect with other caregivers over the internet. The most recent threads were usually months old and nobody ever answered my queries. I've never enjoyed social media, so that eliminated Facebook groups as an option.

The wide array of types of this disease created another complication: written descriptions of experiences rarely related to my immediate issues. There are so many varieties of

Alzheimer's that it was difficult to learn what to expect. I found a few books written by caregivers and they were very helpful, but I never did locate what I wanted most: a local group where I could connect with fellow caregivers, ask questions, and find answers and support.

During the Manor years, we were fortunate to have the support of professional staff with years of memory-care experience. The doctors, nurses and CNAs were respectful of my recommendations and held regular care conferences with me. On a few occasions, I met other caregivers in the parking lot and found them feeling just as isolated and hungry for information about what to expect as I was. I helped one caregiver with the suggestion that his family set up a trust as we had done. He later thanked me profusely.

When I was young, anyone over the age of sixty-five was likely to be a little forgetful. Most people didn't live long enough to be diagnosed with Alzheimer's. Now it's common to see folks like me in their eighties enjoying a full life, but it's also common to see many falling victim to this most debilitating of ailments, while their children in their sixties become their caregivers.

Those caregivers have become the forgotten soldiers in the ever-expanding battle against Alzheimer's. If you count the number of nursing facilities in a thirty-mile radius of your home and figure fifty rooms each and about half of their patients having memory loss, that equals many thousands of caregivers in the U.S. desperately seeking information, guidance and support. Many caregivers struggle with their own health issues and risk their longevity by their dedication to their loved ones. Others, sadly, give up and don't even visit anymore once their family member moves into a long-term care facility.

The number of caregivers will continue to multiply as life expectancy keeps rising while there is little progress toward finding a cure for Alzheimer's. A solution is long overdue.

I hope that in the near future, there will be more effective treatments for this debilitating disease, along with greater emphasis on local support-group meetings for caregivers throughout the country—including in rural areas and small towns. This could be organized under the guidance of an experienced organization such as the Alzheimer's Association. The effort could be assisted by national and state health departments and health insurance companies. The result would be an effective network of local support groups with professional overview, available to America's thousands of devoted caregivers.

Chapter Seven: Legal Concerns

When you become a caregiver for a loved one with Alzheimer's, it's a good idea to seek advice from an attorney and a financial planner. These two professionals will be an important source of guidance and support throughout your caregiving journey. If you don't yet have an attorney and a financial planner, now is the time to hire them. Ask close friends and relatives for referrals to trusted, experienced professionals in your area. Look for an attorney who specializes in elder-care law in your state.

It's essential that you have the legal authority to make important decisions in the best interest of your loved one, who will be unable to make those decisions for themselves. This legal authorization may be spelled out in a trust, a will, a power of attorney, or a court order. Creating these documents and plans as soon as possible will give you the peace of mind and the legal authority you need to be an effective caregiver.

There will be many decisions that come up, large and small: medications, medical procedures, finances, religious preferences, visitors, resuscitation possibilities, end-of-life decisions and a host of other issues. You need legal documents that spell out your ability to use your loved one's financial resources to provide for their needs and wishes. Without this authority, you may be reduced to the legal status of a visitor.

The following is a list of legal documents you may need to provide to medical facilities, insurance companies, or local courts. If you are the spouse of the Alzheimer's patient, you will also need your own documents, along with a copy of your marriage license. If you or the patient are immigrants, you will also need citizenship or legal residence documents.

For admission to a nursing care facility, you will need the patient's...

- Photo ID
- Heath insurance card
- Medicare card
- Social Security card
- Birth certificate
- Proof of veteran status (if applicable)
- Record of any public assistance received in-state or out-of-state

To activate an existing legal trust, you will need all of the above plus...

- Any pending lawsuits that could benefit the patient
- Any one-time payments in the past 60 days (such as insurance, awards, compensation, lottery winnings, etc.)
- Any tax refunds received in the past year
- Deeds for all real estate owned by the patient and/or spouse: home, vacation properties, oil leases, cemetery plots, etc.
- Property tax bills for the current year
- Titles and values for any vehicles owned by the patient and/or spouse: cars, trucks, motorcycles, RVs, ATVs, boats, farm equipment, etc.
- Lease agreements for any leased vehicles

- Statements for: bank or investment accounts, retirement account, IRA, 401K, stocks, bonds, long-term care insurance
- Income records for salaries, pensions, social security, rental or loan income

- Mortgage statement
- Homeowners insurance statement and utility bills
- Any large gifts or loans of money, vehicles, property, cash, etc. in the last 5 years
- Pre-paid funeral documents and value

This list is intended to provide a basic overview for new caregivers. The documents required will vary depending on the laws in your state and the policies of the long-term care facility you choose. Please consult your attorney and financial advisor for the most accurate, up-to-date local information for your particular situation.

Chapter Eight: Choosing a Care Facility

It's highly recommended that you take the time to tour the long-term care facilities in your area *before* you need their services. Planning ahead will help reduce your stress if you find yourself facing an unexpected medical crisis. Even if your loved one with Alzheimer's doesn't need a long-term care facility right now, having a place in mind will make things less stressful if and when that day arrives.

You can start with a simple internet search for long-term care facilities in your area. Visit their websites and create a list of the places that most appeal to you. Then call to schedule an in-person tour at each of your top choices.

Each facility will have an admissions officer, who is your first contact. That person will offer you a roster of their staff and an outline of their floor plan, which should include areas for physical therapy, dining, entertainment activities, rest rooms and staff work areas.

Make sure the facility is licensed by your state. State licensing assures that standards of medical care, staff qualifications, diet and nutrition standards, cleanliness, security, health, safety, and discrimination guidelines are met.

There should also be security protocols in place. The first time I visited Sylvia indoors at the Manor, I was surprised to discover that I could not simply push the exit door open to leave. A digital code, which changes daily, is required to leave the building, and a sign-in procedure is required to enter. This protects any residents who might wander off, and ensures that everyone who wishes to enter the facility has a reason for visiting. You may also hear fire alarms on a regular basis, as fire drills are required. These are all good signs of a facility that makes patient safety a priority.

Here are some questions to consider as you evaluate the facilities in your area...

- The most important question: does the facility accept the Medicaid, Medicare, or long-term care insurance the patient has? If not, cross it off your list.
- Is the entire place, inside and out, well maintained and clean?
- Are the exterior, grounds, and interior design of the building pleasing? Does it feel warm and welcoming? Look for a place that feels more like a home than an office building.
- Are there flowers, trees and plants outside and are they well maintained? When your loved one is able to be outdoors, a pleasant garden can help reduce anxiety and encourage relaxation.
- Is the staff dressed appropriately? Are they welcoming and forthcoming with information?
- Are there regularly scheduled activities for patients, such as crafts, games, musical performances, and outings or other special events? Live music can be especially enjoyable for Alzheimer's patients.
- Will there be regular care conferences scheduled, to give you updates on your loved one's treatments, medications, doctor visits, changing behaviors and any issues you want to discuss?

- How does the facility handle billing, reimbursements for insurance, and payments for residents' charges?
- How is laundry managed? What personal clothing and decorating items are allowed?
- Are services like hair styling, manicures and pedicures available? How are these scheduled and paid for?
- Does the facility support special ceremonies for veterans? Some will arrange a small color-guard ceremony and presentation of a flag when a veteran enters the hospice phase.
- What are the policies and procedures regarding visits from professionals, such as medical specialists, chaplains, lawyers?
- How does the facility handle agitated patients? How do they handle a patient who sleepwalks or one who likes to wander around the building? Some facilities require that the caregiver or family hire and pay separately for a 24/7 attendant to sit with a difficult-to-manage patient when family members cannot be present.

Chapter Nine: Working with Your Care Facility

When your loved one with Alzheimer's moves into a long-term care facility, your caregiving role enters a new phase. Here is my best advice to help you maneuver successfully through this important, and challenging, transition:

- The facility will schedule regular care conferences for you with the staff members responsible for your loved one's daily care. These meetings provide a valuable opportunity to get up-to-date information and resolve any issues that may arise. You should be familiar with all of your loved one's prescriptions, and come prepared with a list of any problems that you want to correct.

- When visiting your loved one, always show respect and appreciation to the nurses and the entire staff. I found them to be consistently professional and deserving of repeated thanks for jobs well done. Unfortunately, I witnessed more than one incident of flagrant disrespect shown by other visitors. There is never any reason to insult the residents, fellow visitors, or staff members. A negative attitude and toxic behavior can only detract from the care your loved one receives at the hands of the disrespected staff.

- You may find that well-meaning friends and acquaintances like to share their opinion with you that a nursing home is purgatory. Don't hesitate to correct their mistaken idea and explain that modern long-term care facilities provide dedicated, skilled, loving care to their patients.

- Decorate your loved one's room with items that reflect their lifelong hobbies and interests. Favorite photographs, artwork, family pictures, mementoes, and religious symbols may bring them comfort and stimulate pleasant memories. Flourishing plants are always welcome. A bird feeder outside their window can provide enjoyment. A radio, CD or DVD player can provide music and entertainment.

- Install a hook (a removable 3M Command Hook works well) on the outside of the door where you can hang seasonal decorations, cheerful garden flags, or thank-you notes to the staff for their loving care.

- The facility will allow you to provide clothing, blankets, and pillows. To maximize your loved one's comfort and well-being, these should be rotated seasonally.

- To prevent items from getting lost in the laundry, use iron-on labels to identify your loved one's belongings by name and room number. You can order custom iron-on labels from Amazon at affordable prices. There may also be an option to take the laundry home and do it yourself, if you prefer.

- You may not be a dietitian or a nutrition authority, but you very likely know your loved one's food allergies and preferences. Take an active role in placing meal-order tickets. I found this to be difficult to manage because of the timing of those tickets and the timing of my visits, but try to communicate with the kitchen staff as needed.

- The facility may offer an in-house bank account where you can deposit funds to pay for personal services such as hair styling and manicures.
- Transportation is usually available for off-site appointments or visits, if your loved one is well enough to travel. Residents can also be taken to religious services or home to visit family.
- Recreational events and religious services may be provided on-site. Most facilities are open to visiting clergy.
- Be aware that you may experience burn-out due to the ever-increasing demands on your time and endurance. I witnessed many long-term residents who never seemed to have a single visitor, let alone a devoted caregiver. To avoid such a dismal outcome, it's essential to set aside time to care for your own well-being.
- Take time to enjoy your hobbies, your friends, and your family. Remove any guilt for your indulgence. Find a substitute visitor for a few days. Take a vacation. Remodel a room. Buy yourself a treat. Make a day just for you. You've earned a break. Taking some time to renew your strength and refresh your spirit will only enhance your ability to care for your loved one.

I pray that God will wrap His loving arms around all who provide care for those who cannot care for themselves. May you be blessed on your caregiving journey.

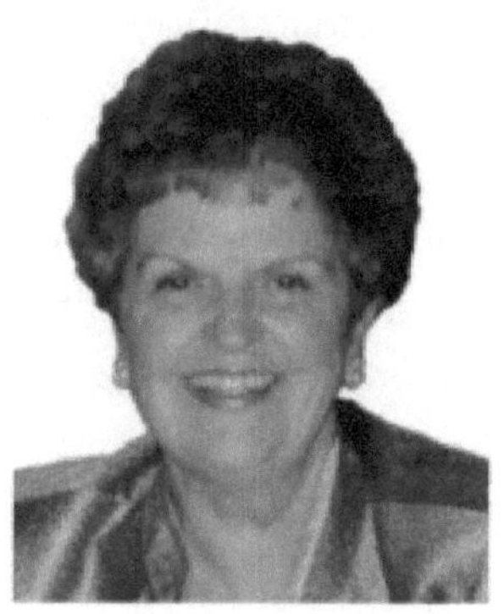

A Remembrance of Sylvia

Sylvia Thacker passed away peacefully in January 2024 at the age of 85 after a long journey with Alzheimer's. She was the beloved wife of her devoted husband Bob for 64 years, the beloved mother of son Gregg and daughter Shelly, and the beloved grandmother of two granddaughters.

Born in a small town in Ontario, Canada, Sylvia pursued all three of the careers that were open to women in that era: she worked as a teacher in a one-room schoolhouse; as a secretary in her step-father's car dealership; and later became a nurse with a particular talent and love for working with the elderly. After her youngest child left the nest, Sylvia left nursing to make her lifelong dream of opening a restaurant come true.

The Sweet Afton Tea Room, a British Victorian restaurant and bakery, won rave reviews from the media and customers alike, and was honored as one of the top ten restaurants in Metro Detroit by the *Detroit News*. She eventually sold Sweet Afton when she and Bob moved Up North to a picturesque town on the shores of Lake Huron to enjoy their retirement.

Sylvia loved baking, watching "I Love Lucy," collecting and reading vintage books, and Elvis. She was a member of Mensa, a loyal pen-pal to friends near and far, and was rarely without a companion cat in her life.

She would be proud that her lifelong love of music lives on in her granddaughters. Sylvia's voice shines through in every note her granddaughters play and sing.

Sylvia had a special fondness for the British Royal Family, a proper cup of tea, and all things English. It makes us smile to imagine her in Heaven now, her health and all her memories restored...perhaps sipping a cuppa with Her Majesty.

Rest in peace in the arms of your Savior, dearest Mum. We will love you and remember you forever.

- Shelly Thacker Meinhardt
January 2024

Sweet Afton Scottish Shortbread Recipe

Makes: 80 cookies (each about 1-1/2" square)

Preheat oven to 325 degrees Fahrenheit

Ingredients

- 4 cups all-purpose flour
- 1 cup white sugar
- 1 pound (4 sticks) salted cold butter of the best quality, cut into small cubes

Method

Place all ingredients in a medium or large bowl. With clean, warm hands, sit down and work ingredients together until the dough is well incorporated and has the consistency of soft ice-cream. This will take 30-45 minutes to reach the proper blend...so be patient.

On a regular, full-size cookie sheet with sides, pull off chunks of dough and place all over to roughly fill the pan. Your goal here is to make an even layer from side to side. Use the heels of your hands to press the dough down *gently* but firmly until the entire pan is covered evenly. Using a fork, prick holes in the dough all up and down the pan, making sure that the tines go all the way through to the cookie sheet itself. You can do this randomly, or make a pattern if you wish, but make sure you create lots of little holes across the dough. This keeps the shortbread from buckling.

Bake in pre-heated oven at 325 degrees for 20 to 25 minutes (until *very lightly* brown). Remove from oven, cool 5 minutes, and cut immediately into size you desire (about 1½" square). Store in tightly covered tin or container. This shortbread keeps well...in fact it gets even better with age!

This was the most popular cookie served at the Sweet Afton Tea Room. Enjoy!

Sweet Afton Scones Recipe

Makes: 2 Dozen Scones (about 2" each)

Preheat oven to 400 degrees Fahrenheit

Ingredients

- 4 cups all-purpose flour
- 4 tablespoons white sugar
- 6 teaspoons baking powder
- 8 tablespoons butter, cold, cut into small cubes
- 4 large eggs
- 2/3 cup buttermilk
- 3/4 cup currants
- Cream for brushing tops
- Coarse sugar for sprinkling

Method

In a medium bowl, stir together flour, sugar, and baking powder. Cut in cold butter until coarse crumbs form. Mix in currants.

In a measuring cup, mix together lightly whisked eggs and buttermilk.

Form a well in the dry ingredients, pour in the liquid and stir quickly.

Turn out the dough on a floured board, then knead gently until it just sticks together. Pat out the dough 1" thick and cut with round 2" biscuit cutter. Place scones on a baking sheet lined with baking parchment.

Brush tops with cream and sprinkle with coarse sugar.

Bake in pre-heated oven at 400 degrees for 10-12 minutes until lightly browned.

At the Sweet Afton Tea Room, scones were served warm with Devon cream and jam or lemon curd. Enjoy!

About the Author

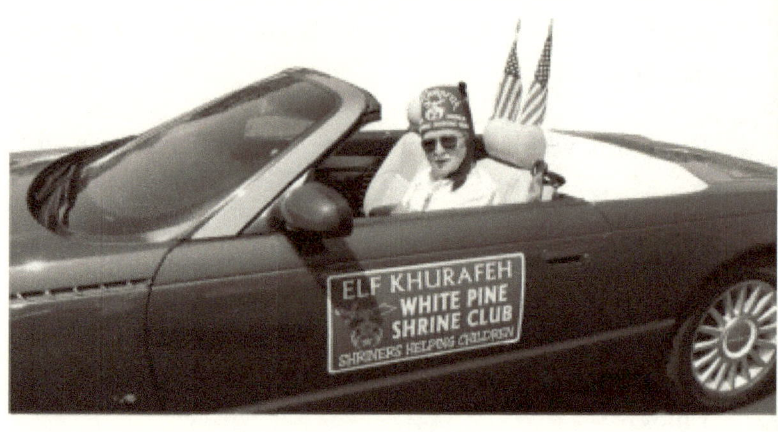

Robert D. Thacker enjoyed 42 years as a creative contributor to automotive design, beginning as a clay sculptor followed by 26 years in model development management. He especially enjoyed writing technical manuals and financial justifications. In retirement, his love of old cars continues to flourish and he maintains and shows vintage Fords in parades and at local festivals. With his keen interest in history, he has contributed numerous articles and photos to collector car magazines.

Robert is an active member of three fraternal organizations which provide college scholarships for young people and support for children suffering from birth defects, burn injuries, and dyslexia. He particularly enjoys blending his charitable work with his love of vintage cars, as seen in the photo above.

Copyright

This memoir is a truthful recollection of actual events in the author's life. Some conversations have been recreated. The names and details of some individuals and businesses have been changed to respect their privacy. This book is not intended as a substitute for professional medical or legal advice. It is not meant to be used, nor should it be used, to diagnose or treat any medical or psychological condition. Readers are advised to consult their own medical and legal advisors whose responsibility it is to determine the condition of, and best treatment plan for, the reader. The content presented herein is based on the author's perspective and interpretation of the subject matter. Neither the publisher nor any associated parties shall be held responsible for any consequences arising from the opinions or interpretations expressed within this book.

~ ~ ~

Publishing History
First edition published by Summit Avenue Books
Copyright © 2024 by Robert D. Thacker
Version 7.3.24

~ ~ ~

All rights reserved. No part of this book, except in the case of brief quotations embodied in critical articles or reviews, may be reproduced in any form by any means, including information

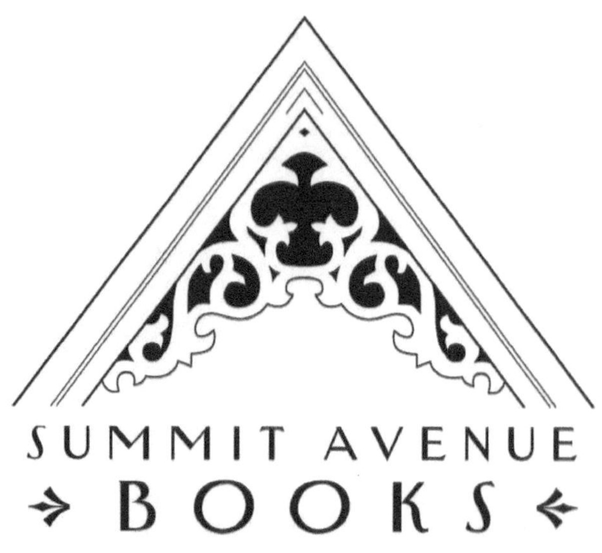

About the Publisher

Summit Avenue stretches for five remarkable miles through the heart of Minnesota's capital, St. Paul. Lined with restored Victorian mansions, this elegant boulevard has been the city's most sought-after address since before the Civil War. Once home to lumber barons, railroad tycoons, and authors like F. Scott Fitzgerald and Sinclair Lewis, Summit Avenue today is still a place for those who believe in their dreams and work hard to achieve them. Summit Avenue Books publishes fiction and non-fiction by some of today's best independent authors.